# Slim Down Revolution

Simplifying weight loss, Be lectin free,
Unleash your inner health.

Antwan L. McElroy

# COPYRIGHT MESSAGE

Slim Down Revolution

# TABLE OF CONTENT

**Introduction**

**Chapter 1: Stand Your Adversary**
- Debunk Common Diet Myths And Misconceptions
- Problems With The Present Day Diet

**Chapter 2: Navigating The Diet Jungle**
- Lectins Roaming Free
- Developing A Positive Relationship With Food And Your Body

**Chapter 3: Transform Your Habits**
- Knights Of Fat Loss
- Discovering The Secrets Of Boosting Fat

**Chapter 4: Sustainable Weight Loss**
- Role Of Healthy Habits And Lifestyle
- Reaping Rewards And Celebrating Success

**Conclusion**

# INTRODUCTION

Greetings on your voyage to a happier, healthier version of yourself! This book is your road map to reaching your weight reduction objectives and forming long-lasting habits for a healthier lifestyle. We are aware that losing weight entails more than just packing on the pounds; it also involves enhancing general health and wellbeing.

So let's set off on this adventure together and explore all of the opportunities that await like Emily.

For her vibrant green eyes and her infectious laughter, she carried a heavy burden. Emily had always struggled with her weight, often feeling self-conscious and unhappy with her appearance.

One day, as she strolled through the local bookstore, she stumbled upon a book titled " Slim Down Revolution" Intrigued by the colorful cover and the promise of a healthier lifestyle, Emily decided to give it a chance. Little did she know, this book would change her life in ways she never imagined.

As she delved into the pages of "Slim Down Revolution," Emily discovered a whole new world of nutritious recipes, exercise routines, and most importantly, self-love and acceptance. The book emphasised the importance of nourishing her body with wholesome, green foods, and seeking a leaner physique as a byproduct of a healthy lifestyle, rather than an obsession.

Motivated by the book's empowering message, Emily resolved to implement its teachings into her life. She started by visiting local farmers' markets and filling her kitchen with an array of vibrant, fresh fruits and vegetables.

With these colourful ingredients, she experimented with flavorful new recipes, revelling in the joy of creating nourishing meals that satisfied her body and soul. Each day, she dedicated time to exploring the picturesque trails surrounding her town, reveling in the beauty of nature and embracing physical activity as a source of strength and joy.

As she immersed herself in this new lifestyle, Emily found herself shedding not only unwanted weight but also the burdens of self-doubt and negativity. She revelled in the newfound energy that coursed through her body, propelling her to embrace each day with optimism and vitality. Her vibrant green eyes sparkled with a newfound inner light, and her infectious laughter echoed through the town, spreading joy and inspiration to those around her.

Emily's transformation became a beacon of hope for others struggling with their own wellness journeys. People admired her renewed confidence and admired the radiant glow that now emanated from within her. She became a source of encouragement, sharing her story and the lessons she gleaned from "Slim Down Revolution" with anyone eager to embark on their own path to wellness.

The once self-conscious and burdened Emily had blossomed into a vibrant, spirited individual who embodied the wisdom and joy found within the pages of "Slim Down Revolution." Her journey was no longer solely about achieving a certain appearance, but about embracing a holistic, nourishing lifestyle that resonated deep within her being.

And so, Emily's story continued to unfold, an inspiring testament to the transformative power of self-love, healthy living, and the profound impact of a single book's message. Emily, with her luminous green eyes and infectious laughter, had become a living testament to the profound impact of embracing a healthy life.

## WHY THIS BOOK

This book is your ultimate guide to achieving a healthier, fitter, and more confident version of yourself. Get ready to embark on a revolutionary journey towards a slimmer and more vibrant you!

1. Discover the Secrets:
In "Slim Down Revolution," we unveil the well-kept secrets to successful weight loss and body transformation. This book is packed with

scientifically proven strategies, expert advice, and practical tips that will empower you to take control of your health and reshape your body.

2. Revolutionize Your Approach:
Say goodbye to fad diets and temporary fixes. "Slim Down Revolution" revolutionizes the way you approach weight loss by providing you with a sustainable and long-term solution. It focuses on creating healthy habits, nourishing your body, and embracing a positive mindset that will lead to lasting results.

3. Personalized Plan:
No two individuals are the same, and that's why "Slim Down Revolution" emphasizes the importance of a personalized approach. Discover how to tailor your nutrition, exercise, and lifestyle choices to fit your unique needs and preferences. This book will guide you in creating a customized plan that works specifically for you.

4. Empowering Mindset:
Achieving your weight loss goals is not just about physical changes; it's also about cultivating a positive and empowering mindset. "Slim Down Revolution" provides you with the tools to overcome self-doubt, stay motivated, and develop a healthy relationship with your body. Unlock the power of your mind and transform your life.

5. Sustainable Results:
Forget about quick fixes and yo-yo diets. "Slim Down Revolution" focuses on sustainable results that will last a lifetime. By implementing the principles outlined in this book, you will not only shed unwanted pounds but also improve your overall well-being, boost your energy levels, and enhance your self-confidence.

Are you ready to join the "Slim Down Revolution" and embark on a transformative journey towards a healthier and happier you? This book is your roadmap to success, providing you with the knowledge, guidance, and inspiration you need to achieve your weight loss goals. Get ready to revolutionize your body, mind, and life. It's time to unleash the power of transformation!

# A GUIDE ON HOW TO USE THIS BOOK"

This guide is designed to help you navigate and make the most of the valuable information contained within the book. Whether you're looking to shed a few pounds, adopt a healthier lifestyle, or embark on a transformative weight loss journey, this book is here to support you. Let's dive into how you can effectively use this book to achieve your goals.

1. Familiarize Yourself with the Content:
Start by familiarizing yourself with the structure and content of the book. Take a moment to read the table of contents and get an overview of the chapters and sections. This will give you a sense of the topics covered and help you plan your reading journey.

2. Set Clear Goals:
Before diving into the book, it's important to set clear goals for yourself. Determine what you want to

achieve through the "Slim Down Revolution" and write down your objectives. This will help you stay focused and motivated throughout the process.

3. Read and Absorb:

As you read each chapter, take your time to absorb the information. Pay attention to the author's insights, tips, and strategies. Take notes if necessary and highlight key points that resonate with you. Remember, knowledge is power, and the more you absorb, the better equipped you'll be to implement the principles outlined in the book.

4. Create an Action Plan:

Once you've gained a solid understanding of the book's content, it's time to create an action plan. Identify the specific steps and changes you need to make in your daily life to align with the principles discussed. Break down your goals into smaller, manageable tasks and create a timeline for implementation.

5. Implement and Track Progress:
Put your action plan into motion and start implementing the strategies outlined in the book. Stay consistent and track your progress along the way. Regularly assess your achievements, make adjustments if necessary, and celebrate your successes.

6. Seek Support and Accountability:
Embarking on a weight loss or lifestyle transformation journey can be challenging. Seek support from friends, family, or online communities who share similar goals. Consider finding an accountability partner who can help keep you motivated and on track.

By familiarizing yourself with the content, setting clear goals, absorbing the information, creating an action plan, implementing strategies, and seeking support, you'll be well on your way to a successful slim down revolution. Remember, the power to transform your life lies within you, and this book is here to guide and inspire you every step of the way.

# CHAPTER 1

## STAND YOUR ADVERSARY

Losing weight is difficult for the majority of us. In fact, it's frequently simply impossible because weight loss adversaries lurk around every turn. Even if you follow a healthy diet and exercise routine religiously, those stubborn pounds might be difficult to lose.

If you've struck a snag in your weight-loss journey, it's essential to uncover any lurking opponents that are impeding your progress. The good news is that once identified, these impediments are simple to remove. Even identifying just one can have a significant impact on your weight loss objectives.

1. Refined Carbohydrates

You must consume carbohydrates! If you consume the correct carbs, they're not the enemy that the media portrays them to be.

A sufficient amount of the right carbs provides energy to your body and brain.

You should incorporate complex carbohydrates in your diet (such as brown rice, oats, quinoa, and veggies), which are good providers of energy and nourishment. However, avoid simple or processed carbs, which promote obesity, high blood sugars, and chronic inflammation. Most processed snack items and anything produced with white flour or sugar are examples.

Dehydration is number two.
A cactus in a pot next to a glass of water; the link between dehydration, weight loss, and incontinence

You've definitely heard about drinking to prevent fluid retention, but did you know it also has an effect on weight loss? Dehydration slows down many chemical events in the body, including fat burning. Even if you're dieting and exercising, a lack of hydrating fluids prevents you from burning fat.

While dehydration might be a major obstacle, it's also one of the most easily overcome weight loss enemies. But remember that the commonly advised 64 ounces of water each day are only guidelines. Find your optimal fluid intake that keeps you feeling good without making frequent trips to the bathroom. Most people need more (decaffeinated) hydrating fluids than this.

## 3. Overindulgent eating

It's likely that you've heard—and it makes sense—that you should wait to serve seconds. Actually, it takes your brain twenty minutes to register fullness in your stomach and to send the appropriate signal. Therefore, don't be too ready to seek out additional food even if you feel satisfied after your usual piece.

When you eat past the point at which you realize you're full, you are overeating. Consuming food to this degree puts pressure on other organs in your stomach. This makes you feel uncomfortable and full, which usually makes you regret it. "Gah! My mistake was eating too much.

Even worse, overindulging causes a calorie surplus as opposed to a calorie deficit. And as everyone knows, consuming excessive amounts of calories eventually causes weight gain. This is because eating too many calories causes fat to accumulate, which exacerbates obesity.

4. Overindulgence in Sodium

This one might surprise even the most seasoned dieters. It's not just about consuming unhealthy meals or retaining fluids. Researchers have shown that one of the most harmful enemies of weight loss is salt. It has been demonstrated to enlarge fat cells. Ouch!

Although the daily requirement of salt for your body is just 14 teaspoons (575 mg), most people consume 20 times that amount. Whichever diet you decide on, for best health and weight loss, limit your daily sodium consumption to 1500–2000 mg. It is recommended by the American Heart Association to consume fewer than 1500 mg daily.

Recall that you should restrict not only the amount of table salt you consume, but also the amount of processed foods you eat, as they are often high in sodium. Read the labels, please!

5. Lack of Sleep
Hormones linked to appetite can rise when sleep is lacking.

Deprivation of sleep also greatly hinders weight loss. A solid rest is pivotal for weight loss. You can exercise every day and eat nothing, yet your body will adamantly refuse to lose weight. Rather, sleep deprivation slows your metabolism and puts your body in survival mode, which leads to fat conservation.

Even worse, not getting enough sleep increases cortisol, the stress hormone, and hunger hormones. In summary, weight gain and sleep deprivation are strongly correlated. To overcome this obstacle to weight loss, get at least 7-8 hours of sleep every night.

But listen to your body; you could need more, particularly if you have particular health issues.

6. Excessive Stress

Stress manifests itself in a variety of ways.While you may sense the stress of a looming deadline, it is easy to underestimate the impact of prolonged emotional stress. High stress levels are a major cause of halted weight loss and even weight gain, whether you live under the weight of a high-pressure job or a challenging personal situation.

Chronic high stress, including sleep deprivation, raises cortisol levels, which slows or prevents fat burning. The good news is that if you address the underlying issue, whether through management techniques or a change in situation, the weight will often melt away, as long as you keep to a healthy eating plan.

7. Stress Consumption

Eating to relieve anxious emotions rather than hunger is one of the most prominent opponents of weight loss. Most people seek unhealthy foods high in fat, sugar, and calories during times of severe stress.

However, there is science behind these decisions. Junk food and processed foods contain high levels of dopamine and other feel-good chemicals, so you may come to rely on them to make you feel better.

If you're craving comfort food, try an apple with peanut butter instead of sweets, or unsweetened Greek yogurt with stevia and berries instead of ice cream.

## 8. Caloric Drinks

Two big glasses of cola; Drinking sugary beverages raises thirst and adds calories without providing nutritious value.

Drinking your calories means you're ingesting a lot of sugar, which will swiftly flow through your system and increase your hunger for more food or drink. Fruit juice includes concentrated amounts of natural sugar, far more than a serving requires.

This means you're consuming more calories than if you simply ate a slice of fruit. And, of course, soda is high in sugar and contains no nutritious benefit. Avoid sodas entirely and replace them with flavored, unsweetened seltzer water.

If you wish to drink fruit juice, make sure to count it as part of your daily calorie consumption. However, if you want to obtain more of your calories from food and feel fuller for longer, choose fresh or frozen fruit over juices.

9. Chronic Inflammation

Long-term inflammation causes insulin resistance, which means that your body produces more insulin to lower blood sugar levels. However, insulin is also a fat-storing hormone that stimulates the formation of new fat cells. The extra fat is typically accumulated around the abdomen, creating belly fat and raising your risk of several health concerns.

Inflammation can be reduced by obtaining enough rest, lowering stress, and consuming an anti-inflammatory diet.

## 10. Food Triggers

You usually think of cookies, cakes, potato chips, French fries, and doughnuts when you think of weight loss adversaries like trigger foods. These foods contain a lot of fat, sugar, salt, and calories. And because trigger foods increase the previously mentioned feel-good neurotransmitters, you are more prone to binge on them and overeat.

However, most of the time, it is possible to pass on trigger foods. When you start eating more complex carbs, less sugar, and more protein and fiber, your cravings for trigger foods will gradually subside.

This isn't to say you can't indulge in your favorite food on occasion, but it will be more of a choice rather than a compulsion.

## 11. Sedentary Way of Life

First person perspective from a person in bed with a remote and channel surfing; Dieting without physical activity is unlikely to produce the intended benefits.

You're fighting an uphill battle if you're attempting to reduce weight but don't move much during the day. Simply walking 10,000 steps or more per day and making an effort to move or be active will significantly aid in weight loss, especially if you follow the other suggestions and eat a nutritious diet.

However, if you need more aid with calorie restriction, structured activity such as gym exercises, a regular walking routine, a yoga class, or an aerobics class would most certainly benefit you. If you're having trouble reducing your food intake further, exercise can help you boost your calorie deficit.

Activity and exercise also help to enhance your metabolism and ability to burn fat.

12. Rapid Weight Loss

A crash diet is one that severely restricts calories, which has an impact not only on your overall health but also on your metabolism. Even if you do lose some weight, it takes relatively little to regain it once you resume eating.

It is preferable to eat the proper foods at the right times to encourage healthy weight gain and maintain your metabolism running smoothly.

Crash dieting is not the same as intermittent fasting, which restricts calories for a brief period of time and can help some people lose weight.

## DEBUNK COMMON DIET MYTHS AND MISCONCEPTIONS

It's easy to get lost in a sea of weight reduction advice in the internet age, much of which is based on popular myths and misconceptions. If you've been battling to lose weight, it's critical to separate fact from fantasy. In this post, we'll debunk some of the most common weight reduction myths and give you evidence-based truths to help you control your weight successfully.

Myth 1: Crash diets are the most effective way to lose weight quickly. Crash diets can be harmful to your health and metabolism in the long run. Rapid weight loss is frequently associated with muscle loss and dietary deficits. Weight loss that is sustainable is progressive, safe, and supports your total well-being.

Myth 2: In order to lose weight, you must skip meals. Fact: Skipping meals is unhealthy. It lowers your metabolism and may cause you to overeat later throughout the day. To keep your metabolism functioning, eat fewer, more balanced meals throughout the day.

Myth 3: Carbohydrates Are the Enemy Carbohydrates are not your adversary; they are your body's major source of energy. Choose complex carbs such as healthy grains and veggies while keeping portion quantities in check.

Myth 4: Spot Reduction Is Effective Fact: You cannot lose fat from a specific location by exercising on it.
Overall fat loss is achieved by creating a calorie deficit through food and exercise.

Myth 5: All Calories Are Created Equal The truth is that not all calories are created equal. Calorie quality is important. When opposed to empty calories from sugary snacks, nutrient-dense, complete foods deliver more satiety and improved overall health.

Myth 6: You Should Avoid Strength Training Fact: Strength training is an important part of losing weight. It promotes the development of lean muscle, which increases metabolism and aids in fat loss. Incorporate it into your workout program.

Myth 7: There is no gain without pain. Exercising to the point of pain is not required. Workouts that are consistent and gradual are essential. To avoid injury, pay attention to your body and avoid overexertion.

Myth 8: Weight Loss Supplements Work Like Magic Weight loss supplements are not a miracle cure. The best strategies to reduce weight are to follow a balanced diet and get regular exercise.Before making use of any improvements, speak with your PCP.

Myth 9: The Scale Is the Only Way to Measure Success. Weight loss is about more than simply the number on the scale. Non-scale successes, like increased energy, better sleep, and improved fitness, are also significant signs of success.

Myth 10: Willpower Is Everything Weight loss is not only a matter of willpower. It entails adopting long-term lifestyle adjustments, developing healthy habits, and having a support system to assist you along the way.

Distinguishing between weight loss fact and fiction is critical for your journey to a healthy self. Dispelling these common beliefs can result in more effective, long-term weight management. Remember that success requires a comprehensive strategy that prioritizes total health and well-being over quick cures or shortcuts.

# PROBLEMS WITH THE PRESENT DAY DIET

Weight gain from modern diets is caused by a number of variables. The greater availability of processed and high-calorie meals, for example, makes it easy for people to consume more calories than they expend. Another factor is that many individuals have sedentary lifestyles, which means they do not burn as many calories as they used to. Finally, portion sizes have increased, resulting in higher calorie intake.

Modern diets are also heavy in harmful fats, added sugars, and refined carbs, all of which can lead to weight gain. These foods are frequently less filling and can contribute to overeating. Furthermore, the ease of access to fast food and delivery services makes it easier for consumers to make poor decisions.

To maintain a healthy weight, it is critical to adopt healthier dietary choices and integrate physical activity into your daily routine.
The current diet is dominated by processed, easy meals that are high in calories but deficient in nutrients. This suggests that people are eating more calories than they require, resulting in weight gain.

Furthermore, the sedentary lifestyle that many people now lead, with lengthy hours spent sitting at a desk or in front of a screen, means that they do not burn enough energy to balance off their calorie intake.

Furthermore, many modern diets are high in harmful fats like trans fats, which can raise the risk of heart disease and other health problems. Added sugars, which are commonly present in processed foods and beverages, can also lead to weight gain and have been related to a variety of health issues.

Refined carbs, such as white bread and spaghetti, are another prominent component of modern diets that might contribute to weight gain since they breakdown quickly and induce blood sugar increases.

It is critical to be conscious of our food choices and to make an effort to include more full, healthy foods in our diets. Whole grains, lean meats, and fruits and vegetables are a few examples. Limiting processed and high-calorie foods is also crucial, as is being mindful of portion sizes. Physical activity on a regular basis is also essential for keeping a healthy weight and overall well-being.

We can offset the detrimental impacts of modern diets and live healthier, happier lives by adopting small, lasting modifications to our diets and habits.

Complex things such as health and wellness cannot be reduced to a single isolated number such as how much we weigh or what our body mass index (BMI) is. Weight cannot measure purpose or worth.

Dieting mentality tempts us into thinking "If I am thin, I will be happy" or "If I am not thin, I am a failure," yet it just delivers a fictional short-term solution with long-term damaging physical and mental effects.

Focusing on long-term sustainable solutions for integrating controlled eating habits with a variety of food options will make a complete diet and maintaining a healthy weight a true part of our "way of life."

**Weight and Dietary Fat:**

Diets low in fat have long been hailed as the secret to preserving good health and a healthy weight. But the proof simply isn't there: in the United States, the percentage of calories from fat in people's diets has decreased over the last 30 years, but obesity rates have surged.

Studies conducted on clinical subjects have demonstrated that reducing weight with a low-fat diet is not any easier than with a moderate- or high-fat diet. In fact, study volunteers who follow moderate- or high-fat diets lose the same amount of weight as those who follow low-fat diets, if not somewhat more in certain studies. Low-fat diets do not seem to provide any significant benefits in terms of preventing sickness.

The fact that low-fat diets are usually high in carbohydrates, especially from quickly absorbed meals like white bread and rice, is part of the problem with them.

Diets high in such foods also raise the risk of obesity, diabetes, and heart disease.

The type of fat people eat is considerably more essential than the amount for overall health, and there is some evidence that the same may be true for weight control.

A higher intake of harmful fats —trans fats specifically, but also saturated fats—was associated with weight gain in the Nurses' Health Study, an eight-year study that monitored 42,000 middle-aged and older women, but increased consumption of healthy fats-monounsaturated and polyunsaturated fat-was not.

**Protein and Body Mass Index:**

Higher protein diets appear to provide some weight loss benefits, but only in short-term trials; in longer-term research, high-protein diets appear to perform equally well as other types of diets. Because high-protein diets are typically low in carbohydrate and high in fat, it is difficult to distinguish the benefits of eating a lot of protein from the benefits of eating more fat or less carbohydrate. However, there are a few reasons why consuming a higher percentage of calories from protein may aid in weight loss:

Greater satiety: Compared to eating carbs or fat, those who eat protein feel fuller on less calories.

Greater thermic effect: Compared to other macronutrients, protein requires more energy to process and store, which could lead to increased daily calorie expenditure.

Protein appears to help people retain lean muscle during weight reduction, which can also help enhance the energy-burned side of the energy balance equation.

Diets high in protein and low in carbohydrates enhance blood lipid profiles and other metabolic markers, which may aid in the prevention of heart disease and diabetes. On the other hand, some high-protein foods are healthier than others: Diabetes, colon cancer, and heart disease are all associated with the consumption of red and processed meat.

Substituting almonds, beans, fish, or chicken for red and processed meat appears to reduce the risk of heart disease and diabetes. According to a recent Harvard School of Public Health study, this food regimen may also aid in weight control.

For up to 20 years, researchers studied the eating and lifestyle habits of 120,000 men and women to see how tiny changes contributed to weight increase over time.

Over the course of the trial, people who ate more red and processed meat gained weight--about a pound every four years.

People who ate more nuts gained less weight throughout the course of the study--about a half pound less per four years.

**Carbohydrates and Body Mass Index:**
Lower carbohydrate, greater protein diets may provide some short-term weight loss benefits. However, carbohydrate quality is far more important than carbohydrate quantity when it comes to preventing weight gain and chronic disease.

High-carbohydrate foods include white rice, white bread, white pasta, processed cereals, and other items made from milled, refined grains. Potatoes and fizzy drinks are also bad for you.

In scientific terms, they have a high glycemic index and glycemic load. Such foods generate rapid spikes in blood sugar and insulin, which can trigger hunger and overeating in the short term and, in the long run, raise the risk of weight gain, diabetes, and heart disease.

People who increased their consumption of French fries, potatoes and potato chips, sugary drinks, and refined grains, for example, acquired more weight over time--3.4, 1.3, 1.0, and 0.6 pounds.
In the study on diet and lifestyle modification, the duration was four years, respectively.
People who reduced their use of these items gained less weight.

# CHAPTER 2

## NAVIGATING THE DIET JUNGLE

The diet jungle may definitely get rather wild, but don't worry, I'm here to help you simplify your weight loss journey, unlock your inner wellness, and discover the best version of yourself.

Certain plants contain substances that may be harmful to our health. This method simplifies weight reduction by avoiding or limiting the consumption of these potentially hazardous chemicals. Here are some guidelines to assist you with your journey:

Inform yourself: Learn about the foods that are regarded harmful and why. This will allow you to make more educated eating choices.

Focus on nutrient-rich foods: While this may limit some plant-based foods, it's critical to make sure you're getting enough nutrients.

Experiment with other possibilities: This method may restrict your selections, but it may also open you new opportunity to experiment with different components. Incorporate non-traditional grains such as quinoa or amaranth, try with alternative protein sources such as legumes or lean meats, and experiment with different herbs and spices for taste.

Planning and preparing meals ahead of time will help you remain on track and avoid temptations. Look for meals and meal ideas that follow this phylosophy, and try batch cooking to save time and guarantee you always have healthful alternatives on hand.

Pay attention to your body: Take note of how your body reacts to various foods. Maintain a food journal to monitor any changes in symptoms or energy levels. This will assist you in identifying potential triggers and making required changes to your food regimen.

Consider obtaining help from a healthcare practitioner, licensed dietitian, or nutritionist who is familiar with this approach. They can provide you specific advice, answer your concerns, and make sure you're on the right course to reclaiming your inner health.

Remember that discovering your best self is a one-of-a-kind and individualized adventure. What is effective for one person might not do same for another. Throughout the process, it is critical to be patient, adaptable, and kind to oneself. Be open to trying new things, believe in the power of knowledge, and trust your body's wisdom.

## LECTINS ROAMING FREE

According to a 2019 review in Food and Chemical Toxicology, all plants, as well as grain- and soy-fed animals, contain lectins. According to a 2022 review in the Glycoconjugate Journal, lectins serve as a form of protective strategy for plants in nature because they can be poisonous to insects and act as a natural insecticide. Furthermore, because lectins are not digested, it appears that foods containing lectins would be undesirable to consumers such as animals and humans. Clearly, this is not the case, as lectins are present in many of the foods we consume on a daily basis.

However, according to the same 2022 study, lectin levels in plants fluctuate, and there are several forms of lectins. Raw legumes, such as peas, beans, lentils, soybeans, and peanuts, and whole grains, such as wheat, have the most lectins.

According to a 2019 review in Nutrients, nightshade vegetables (eggplant, tomatoes, peppers, potatoes, and seed spices), squash, and fruit are similarly higher in lectins, prompting many lectin-free diet promoters to recommend avoiding these items.

Foods with Low Lectin Content:
These foods, according to Gundry, are low in lectins and thus suitable for a lectin-free diet.

- Asparagus Avocado

- Brussel sprouts, broccoli, and other cruciferous vegetables
- Sweet potatoes cooked with celery
- Garlic
- Green leafy vegetables
- Mushrooms
- Pasture-raised meats with onions

You will avoid foods that contain lectins (a type of protein) on a lectin-free diet, such as wheat and other grains, dairy products from cows, beans and lentils, practically all fruits, and many vegetables.

Many health specialists have voiced worry that eliminating such a broad range of foods may result in vitamin deficiencies, and the detrimental effects of lectins have not been fully demonstrated.

The lectin-free diet was developed by cardiologist Steven Gundry, MD. He and other diet supporters believe that ingesting lectins can result in weight gain, brain fog, chronic inflammation, poor digestion due to a disordered microbiome, and other negative symptoms.

Naturally, lectin-containing foods will be reduced or avoided when following a lectin-free diet.

However, many typical foods are permitted on the regimen.

Lectin-Containing Foods:

- Meats raised on grains, poultry, or seafood
- The majority of starchy foods, including potatoes, rice, and grains
- Lentils with beans
- Tomatoes, eggplant, and peppers are examples of nightshade vegetables.
- Except for berries in season, fruits
- Dairy items made from cow's milk
- Sugar and sugar-sweetened beverages
- Soy products

The 7-day lectin-free diet is illustrated below, beginning with phase one, which is the most stringent and lasts three days. Keep in mind that this is an example of an unhealthy diet. Before beginning this diet, consult with your doctor.

Day 1: Spinach smoothie with avocado, mint, romaine lettuce, lemon juice, and stevia extract; 3 oz. pastured chicken, sauteed mushrooms and mustard greens with coconut oil; 2 oz. wild-caught salmon, butter lettuce with lemon and olive oil, and steaming asparagus

Day 2: 2 oz. wild-caught halibut with lemon, avocado, and sautéed spinach in coconut oil; spinach smoothie with avocado, mint, romaine lettuce, lemon juice, and stevia extract; cabbage, broccoli, and carrot stir-fry, kimchi

Day 3: Avocado, raw sauerkraut, cooked asparagus; beet greens, avocado, beet, and lemon smoothie; 3 ounces pastured chicken, kale cooked with garlic, lemon, and olive oil

Day four: bok choy, coconut oil, and carrots 3 oz. wild-caught salmon, beet greens, avocado, lemon juice, coconut oil, and walnuts 1 ounce dark chocolate, 3 ounces pastured chicken, shredded cooked Brussels sprouts and raw sauerkraut salad

Day 5: 1 ounce dark chocolate, 1 ounce green mango, walnuts, avocado; leafy greens, hemp protein powder, water, mint, and lemon smoothie; 3 ounces wild-caught cod, raw beet salad with basil and pine nuts

Day 6: Smoothie with coconut milk, almond butter, spinach, and hemp protein powder; avocado and raw beet salad with mustard greens, olive oil, and lemon dressing. 1 ounce dark chocolate, 4 ounces pastured chicken, asparagus, Napa cabbage

Day 7: Gundry MD Bar, 1 ounce dark chocolate, walnuts; avocado and 2 ounces pastured chicken salad with lemon and olive oil dressing on lush greens; 3 ounces wild-caught salmon, hemp seeds, lemon, asparagus.

Tips for Preparing the Lectin-Free Diet

It all comes down to avoiding lectin-containing foods on this diet. Some people may jump immediately into a lectin-free diet, but if you follow Gundry's official regimen, you'll go through three stages.

Phase One: A three-day "cleanse" removes everything save a handful of veggies.
Phase Two: Include all remaining lectin-free foods that have been authorized.
Phase Three (Optional): Limit your animal protein consumption to 4 ounces or less per day and adopt intermittent fasting.

The Benefits of a Lectin-Free Diet

It's unclear whether eliminating lectins from your diet would result in dramatic health benefits such as weight loss, reduced symptoms of chronic inflammation, or improved digestion—but eating a diet low in processed foods may have significant benefits.

Consuming lectins may lower inflammatory response: Some study suggests that consuming lectins may activate an inflammatory response. A study published in the Journal of Immunology in 2017 found a biochemical pathway by which this can occur, hypothesizing that lectins operate as a "danger signal" that increases autoimmune disorders.As a result, lowering or removing lectins may help to reduce inflammation.

Could help with vitamin absorption: Have you ever heard of "anti-nutrients"? Although it may appear to be a contradiction in terms, lectins are occasionally labeled as such because, as they accumulate in the stomach, they might interfere with nutritional digestion and absorption.Eliminating them from your diet may allow your intestines to absorb more critical nutrients.

People suffering from irritable bowel syndrome (IBS) may benefit from the following: Many persons with irritable bowel syndrome discover that certain meals trigger their symptoms, therefore foods high in lectins may increase constipation, diarrhea, bloating, or other IBS symptoms. Some studies suggest that there may be a link between foods high in lectins and those high in FODMAPs (carbohydrates known to induce digestive issues in IBS patients). More research is needed to evaluate how eliminating lectins could help persons with IBS.

Whole foods are prioritized: A lectin-free diet comes with one guarantee: you won't be eating many processed foods. Because of the diet's limits, you'll most likely prepare at home with whole foods like veggies, grass-fed meats, and plant-based lipids.

This might probably be beneficial in a society that consumes much too many calories from manufactured foods. You might even pick up some useful kitchen skills if you have to cook at home.

May reduce illness risk: Studies show that eating more processed foods increases the risk of cardiovascular disease, hypertension, metabolic syndrome, cancer, obesity, and even depression.

It's usually a good idea to eat whole, unadulterated foods whenever feasible, and a lectin-free diet may assist you in doing so.

The Drawbacks of a Lectin-Free Diet

The most significant downside of a lectin-free diet is its restrictive character, which may have negative health consequences.

Limited evidence of effectiveness: Although there is some evidence that lectins may be harmful, there is no agreement among nutrition experts that a lectin-free diet is a beneficial way of treating or avoiding any health condition.

The existing research does not apply to humans: There has been very little research on the effects of lectins on health, and most of it has been done on animals. Furthermore, while some foods (such as raw kidney beans) do contain high enough levels of lectins to cause food poisoning, boiling decreases them to a safe level. (And when was the last time you ate a raw kidney bean?)

It may be difficult to consume enough critical nutrients: Lack of lectins may imply a lack of certain key nutrients. A well-rounded diet with plenty of fiber is especially difficult when you can't eat grains or legumes, and getting plenty of antioxidants is especially difficult when fruits are off the menu. In the long run, a lack of vitamins, minerals, and antioxidants from produce may result in nutrient deficiencies.

Difficult to understand: There's no doubting that the lectin-free diet has a large list of forbidden foods. Adhering to its rigorous limits will almost certainly be difficult, and you may lose out on favorite items that don't make the cut.

May interrupt social eating: Any diet that removes broad categories of foods has the potential to disrupt social eating. You may be unable to participate in the food served when dining out or at parties or events. This can cause worry, frustration, or feelings of isolation.

Many authorized meals are pricey: Although a lectin-free diet encourages the consumption of affordable veggies such as broccoli, carrots, and onions, other recommended items may be costly. Grass-fed meats, goat, sheep, or buffalo dairy products, and high-priced cooking oils like avocado and walnut are not cheap. Before beginning this diet, you should assess whether it is financially possible.

A diet that is overly low in carbs is generally a recipe for lethargy, headaches, mood swings, and other unpleasant side effects.

Constipation may result from a lack of fiber: You may become constipated if you do not consume enough fiber from grains, legumes, fruits, and vegetables.

*Is the Lectin-Free Diet a Good Option for You?*

A lectin-free diet can provide all of the nutrients required for optimum health. You don't have to lose out on the macro and micronutrients you need every day with the range of items on the diet's "yes" list.

A lectin-free diet, on the other hand, can have serious nutritional consequences. Carbohydrates are definitely scarce in this area, so attaining the recommended 45% to 65% of your daily calories from them would be difficult.

Furthermore, because the diet excludes grains, you will fall well short of the 3 ounces of whole grains per day recommended by the 2020 Dietary Guidelines for Americans. Because of the lack of grains (as well as beans, lentils, and a variety of vegetables), it may be difficult to meet your daily fiber goal of 25 grams for women and 38 grams for men.

Furthermore, because fruits are almost entirely excluded from a lectin-free diet, you may struggle to take enough of the nutrients they contain, such as vitamin C, potassium, and folate.

It is feasible to receive all of your nutrients on a lectin-free diet, but it may take some careful planning. On this diet, you're especially likely to miss out on fiber and micronutrients like vitamin C, potassium, and folate.

Some people have reported success with a lectin-free diet for weight loss, increased energy, and improved digestion—but the jury is still out on whether the data supports its use for any health issue. And, because it excludes so many essential items (such as beans, grains, and fruits), this diet is probably not worth following for most people.

If you're thinking about going lectin-free, consider how much you're ready to give up and for what potential benefits. And, as with any diet, ask your doctor or a trained nutritionist before embarking on a lectin-free diet.

Remember that following a long-term or short-term diet may not be necessary for you, and many diets, especially long-term diets, simply do not work.

While we do not support fad diets or unsustainable weight loss approaches, we do give the facts so that you can make an informed decision that best suits your nutritional needs, genetic blueprint, budget, and goals.

If weight loss is your aim, keep in mind that reducing weight isn't always synonymous with being your healthiest self, and there are many other methods to achieve health. Your general health is greatly affected by lifestyle choices, exercise, and sleep patterns, among other things. A balanced diet that works for your lifestyle is the ideal one.

## DEVELOPING A POSITIVE RELATIONSHIP WITH FOOD AND YOUR BODY

In an ideal world, we would eat in accordance with our hunger cues, completely enjoy our meals, and select more healthy foods wherever available. However, this is frequently far more complex than it appears. Because of cultural pressure to appear a specific way, 91% of college-aged women have tried dieting at some point, and 61% of females and 28% of males have experienced disordered eating.

"Eating healthy" refers not just to the food you consume, but also to your relationship with food.

So, what constitutes a healthy relationship with food? A healthy relationship includes relaxed eating, preference over position, and eating with balance and flexibility.

In this context, "relaxed eating" refers to eating in accordance with your hunger signals while acknowledging that these signals may alter depending on your routine, moods, and physical needs. It also implies that eating differently from one day to the next should not be reason for concern, condemnation, or punishment.

**"Preferences"** are foods you prefer to consume, whereas "positions" are inflexible habits and a dread of trying new things.

Thus, "choosing preferences over positions" implies accepting that your preferences may not be appropriate in every scenario and being satisfied to choose from the other available possibilities.

**"Balance"** refers to "everything in moderation," which includes all food groups. There is no need to avoid eating any particular food unless you are doing so for religious or ethical reasons, or unless you have been ordered to do so by a doctor.
"Balance" also entails eating for both pleasure and hunger, as well as avoiding diets (spoiler alert: diets don't work in the first place).

**"Flexibility"** can be summed up as "the absence of strict rules surrounding eating and food habits." This involves doing away with the categories "good/clean food" and "bad/junk food." Some foods are more nutritious than others, but a balanced diet – and, more importantly, a healthy relationship with food – typically includes a wide variety of foods.
In other words, a healthy relationship with food is one in which there is no fixation, restriction, worry, or guilt.

Eating is not a precise science, and tracking calories does not produce cortisol.

Tracking calories and macros (short for macronutrients: carbs, fat, and protein) is popular among bodybuilders and athletes, but it is not required for the typical individual and may be harmful for those with a background with eating disorders.

Intuitive eating is an alternative to tracking your daily intake. Listening to your body, observing how certain meals make you feel differently than others, and eating when you are hungry until you are full are all examples of intuitive eating.
It entails rejecting diet culture, making eating joyful and stress-free, and honoring yourself and your unique requirements.

The 80/20 strategy is the result of a search for a healthy eating regimen that does not involve any calories. The 80/20 approach to eating advises that around 80% of your foods should be minimally processed, plant-focused foods, with the remaining

20% being anything you choose to eat, possibly comfort foods.

Despite the fact that you're consuming 20% less nutritious meals, there's no need to feel guilty or sorrow — comfort foods may really improve your health in an unexpected way!

# CHAPTER 3

## TRANSFORM YOUR HABITS

Create simple behaviours.

Long-term, healthy weight loss necessitates a change in your food and exercise habits. However, many other daily decisions, like as how much time you spend sleeping or accessing the Internet, also have an impact.

The routines suggested here can assist you in reaching your healthy weight-loss goal.

Set short, clear, and attainable goals.

Maybe you want to be the same size you were in high school or when you got married, but go there no more—at least not just yet. Set a more realistic aim of reducing 5% to 10% of your body weight, and allow yourself plenty of time and flexibility to attain that goal, bearing in mind that most people require at least six months to achieve that level of healthy weight reduction. Also, avoid broad goals like "I should eat less at dinner and exercise more." Set targeted and short-term (daily or weekly) goals instead, such as these:

On Sunday, I'll choose a couple dinner recipes and go grocery shopping.
Instead of eating out at least three times next week, I will bring a healthy lunch from home.
On Mondays and Wednesdays, I'll phone a friend and go for a walk after work.

To avoid temptation, I will reduce my exposure to troublesome foods ("stimulus control"), such as storing cookies out of sight in the kitchen.

Every morning, eat breakfast slowly and carefully.

Many folks skip breakfast because they are too busy or are not hungry. To make time for breakfast, try getting up 15 minutes earlier (which also implies going to bed earlier so you don't lose sleep time).

Slow down your eating by putting down your fork or sipping water, coffee, or tea between bites. You should spend at least 20 minutes on each meal, but this may be more practical at your midday or evening meal; choose one to begin. Set a timer to check your progress.

Choose the one that appears to be the most feasible for you and try to stick with it for a week or so. It is critical to include these healthy practices into your daily routine.

Add another once you've gotten the hang of one. Many of these habits will become apparent to you as time passes.

## THE KNIGHTS OF FAT LOSS

Before you begin, it is critical to identify some specific goals that you wish to achieve. Whether it's to lose a certain amount of weight or body fat, or simply to become a healthier person. Making these goals can help you stay motivated and consistent throughout the process.

Another important aspect of transforming your body is developing a comprehensive regimen.
Making long-term changes to your health and lifestyle habits is necessary for successful weight loss.

*How do you make long-term changes?*

Make certain that you are prepared.

Take a moment to ask yourself the following questions to assess your readiness:

Is it possible for me to reduce weight?
Are other pressures causing me to become distracted?
Is it time for me to learn or employ new stress-management techniques?
Do I require more assistance in dealing with stress, either from friends or professionals?

# 1st. NUTRITION

It's difficult to be called Sustain Nutrition and not have nutrition at the heart of your mission. Most people will struggle to mindset, lifestyle, and exercise their way to long-term health and happiness if they do not focus on nutrition.

We feel that most people do not need to weigh their food or track their calories. Most individuals eat too little protein and vegetables during the day and eat too much refined, processed, high-calorie food at night. Those who balance the most of their days well have days with inadequate balance and thereby blow their progress.

As a result, if you can add consistency to your days and weeks, you'll have more success.

People who add more protein and vegetables to their diets (3 palm-sized protein servings per day and 2 fist-sized veg) feel fuller, consume fewer calories, eat less junk, and lose weight.

## 2 - EXERCISE

Exercise will support any fat loss attempts as well as other health-related aims. We deteriorate as we age. We lose muscle, fitness, and mobility; this can be countered by proactively focusing on these things.

But where to begin? This is dependent on your current location.

Option A: If you're not doing anything, DO SOMETHING. Walk, go to the gym, and watch TV on the cross trainer. Simply accomplish more than you are today, and make it pleasurable and sustainable.

Option B1 - If you don't want to modify what you're doing, just keep doing it. Attend more zumba sessions, walk more, and eat your lunch standing up. Anything that requires more energy than you were previously using will get you closer to your objective, but it will not have the same impact as selecting the best technique.

Option B2 - If you're just doing something, do it better. Running or lifting weights will enhance your fitness, strength, and muscle mass if you perform yoga or walk. It's great if you don't want to do that, but there are optimal and inferior alternatives. Most people can get to where they wish to go by engaging in their preferred form of exercise.

Option C - If you are doing ideal exercise (a combination of resistance and cardio training in our perspective), then do it better. Improve your strength and fitness. Keep track of what you're doing and your progress over time. You're guessing if you're not assessing. Use an app or an old-fashioned pen and pad to do more over time.

## 3 - ATTITUDE

If you don't adjust your thinking, the efforts listed above are likely to be part-time and unsuccessful.

The tactics to changing mentality depend on where you are, and this is where coaching comes in handy to unpick how people think. Journaling your thoughts and reflecting on them is an excellent place to start. Is this the whole truth or just your interpretation of it?

We are so eager to believe that we are seeing the world as it is, yet this is not the case. Everything is tainted by our perspective, and the more aware we are of this, the better able we are to respond effectively and adjust our behavior.

Many people emotionally eat, that is, eat for reasons other than hunger, and unless we adjust our thinking, this can lurk in the shadows and undermine the gains made by many people who have lost weight and believe their habits have changed.

## 4 - PERSONALITY

Food is linked to the fact that no man or woman is an island. Do you despise your work, partner, or friends? Are you continually being scrutinized, questioned, and criticized? Do you have a solid support network, or are you struggling on your own?

Are you pessimistic and negative, or do you constantly put others ahead of yourself?

This list demonstrates that there is more to fat loss than simply you. It's not simply what you eat, how much you exercise, and how you think.

We are all parts of a larger mechanism. And if we aren't, that produces problems for us as well!

This frequently reveals some unpleasant truths, but it is for this reason that so many individuals lose and regain weight. Weight loss and health will not be sustained for many people unless we examine our lifestyle.

## DISCOVERING SECRETS OF BOOSTING FAT BURN

Your body stores calories as fat in order to keep you alive and safe. There are numerous gimmicks that claim to increase fat burning, such as working out in the fat-burning zone, spot reduction, and foods or supplements that ostensibly cause you to burn more fat.

Instead of looking for a quick fix that is unlikely to work, discover how to burn fat through a range of sorts of exercise if you want to lower the amount of fat stored in your body. Here's what you should know.

The Fundamentals of Fat Burning
Knowing how your body uses calories for fuel can make a difference in how you approach weight management if you're aiming to minimize your body's fat stores. Fat, carbs, and protein provide energy. The one your body uses for energy depends on the activity you're doing.

The majority of people prefer to get their energy from fat. It may appear that the more fat you can use as fuel, the less fat your body will have. However, using more fat does not automatically result in reducing more fat.

Understanding the best technique to burn fat begins with understanding how your body obtains energy.

High-intensity sports, such as fast-paced running, force the body to rely on carbohydrates for sustenance. The metabolic pathways for breaking down carbohydrates for energy are more efficient than those for fat breakdown.
For longer, slower exercise, fat is used for energy more than carbs.

Consider this: when you sit or sleep, your body is in fat-burning mode. But you probably don't see sitting and sleeping as a technique to lose body fat.

The fundamental line is that just consuming more fat as energy does not imply that you are burning more calories.

This does not necessarily imply that if you want to burn more fat, you should avoid low-intensity exercise. There are particular things you can do to burn more fat, and it all begins with how frequently and for how long you exercise.

Achieve fat loss by incorporating both cardiovascular exercises and strength training into your workout routine.

High-intensity cardio is defined as working at 80% to 90% of your maximal heart rate (MHR). If you're not utilizing heart rate zones, aim for a six to eight on a 10-point scale of perceived exertion. This translates to exercising at a level that seems difficult and leaves you too out of breath to speak in entire phrases.

But you're not sprinting as fast as you possibly can.

Short workouts dispersed throughout the day can provide the same benefits as continuous training. For instance, if a person weighs 150 pounds, they can expect to burn around 341 calories by running at a speed of 6 mph for half an hour. On the other hand, if they choose to walk at a pace of 3.5 mph for the same duration, they would burn approximately 136 calories.

However, the number of calories you can burn isn't the only factor to consider. Too many high-intensity workouts per week can endanger you in a variety of ways.

Workouts of Moderate Intensity
For weight loss, you should probably keep the majority of your cardio sessions in the moderate level. Here are a few examples:

A aerobic machine workout lasting 30 to 45 minutes
A quick stroll
Riding a bike at a moderate speed

Low-Intensity Exercise
Low-intensity exercise is defined as exercise that is less than 60% to 70% of your MHR, or a level three to five on a 10-point perceived effort scale. This degree of intensity is without a doubt one of the most comfortable zones of training, keeping you at a speed that isn't too taxing or difficult.

It entails long, slow activities that you may do all day. Even better, it incorporates things you already enjoy, such as going for a walk, gardening, riding a bike, or stretching gently.

Low-intensity exercise can be done throughout the day by doing an extra lap while shopping, using the stairs, parking farther away from the entrance, and doing more physical duties around the house.

Lift Weights to Lose Weight
Increasing muscle mass by lifting weights and performing other resistance activities can also aid in fat loss.

While many people focus on cardio for weight loss, there's no denying that strength training is an important part of any weight loss regimen. Let me present to you a few benefits of engaging in weight training;
Consume Calories
Maintain Metabolism and Muscle Mass.

# CHAPTER 4

## SUSTAINABLE WEIGHT LOSS

Achieving long-term weight loss is a popular aim, but it can be difficult to achieve in the middle of fad diets and short cures.

Sustainable weight loss is about adopting a healthier lifestyle that you can maintain over time, not about short fixes or drastic tactics.

Setting realistic goals, eating a balanced diet, practicing mindful eating, getting regular exercise, staying hydrated, prioritizing sleep and stress management, recording your progress, and seeking support and accountability will help you achieve long-term weight reduction success. Remember that it's not just about losing weight; it's about living a healthier, happier life.

# ROLE OF HEALTHY HABITS AND LIFESTYLE

Weight loss requires healthy behaviors and a healthy lifestyle. You can improve your general well-being by exercising excellent habits such as eating a well-balanced diet, getting regular exercise, and emphasizing self-care. By incorporating these behaviors into your daily routine, you can develop a lasting and healthy lifestyle that will aid in your weight loss efforts.

Weight loss requires healthy behaviors and a healthy lifestyle. You may lose weight and keep it off for good by adding habits like regular exercise, balanced nutrition, and self-care into your daily routine.

These behaviors assist in increasing your metabolism, controlling cravings, and improving your entire physical and emotional well-being, making it simpler to achieve and maintain a healthy weight. Furthermore, cultivating healthy habits and making lifestyle adjustments might help you avoid a variety of health problems and potentially live a longer life. Overall, they play an important role in obtaining and maintaining a healthy weight.

## FUN ACTIVITIES THAT WORK

### CYCLING

Your bike or cycle demonstrates that a fitness gear does not have to be difficult. Cycling, in addition to being a pleasurable sport, is another technique to maximize calorie and fat burning on days when you don't go to the gym.

Cycling is one of the skills we learn as children. Most of us were proud of our ability to cycle when we were younger, and we should have been. However, it is more than just a recreational hobby. Cycling is a fantastic low-impact aerobic exercise and a good training session for losing weight and abdominal fat.

It's reasonable to question how cycling can help you lose weight.

When it comes to losing weight, we've all wondered how we can burn more calories. Cycling is an excellent activity to consider. Cycling for an hour can help you burn up to 500 calories. Of course, depending on activity and rider weight, the number of calories burned every hour might range from 400 to 1000. According to research, riding in the morning, preferably on an empty stomach, burns fat 20% faster and more effectively.

If you want to attain your goal by riding, the time spent pedaling is critical. Longer rides and uphill rides help you burn calories and lose abdominal fat. A leisurely hour of cycling burns approximately 520 calories. Riding at a high intensity for a prolonged period of time might burn up to 782 calories each hour.

There are gym bikes that automatically track your calories. In general, stationary bikes may make it more difficult to burn calories than real bikes.

Cycling at low to moderate resistance for longer periods of time maintains your heart rate up and fat-burning. It allows you to burn enough calories without gaining bulky muscles. Furthermore, as long as you maintain a calorie deficit with your food and ride your bike regularly, you will be able to drop 500 grams in a week.

Whether you have a little or a lot of weight to lose, a well-planned cycling program can help you burn more calories. Weight loss is as simple as eating correctly and moving more. Cycling and the appropriate meal choices can help you burn up to 500 calories each hour. However, keep in mind that everyone's metabolism is unique. As a result, the rate of calorie burning fluctuates.

This is an important advice. A pre-dawn bike ride is the most enjoyable approach to commence your weight loss. You're probably thinking it's insane to go cycling first thing in the morning with no petrol in your tank. Listen to us out first.

The rationale is that you will begin fasting training, in which your body will use stored fat for energy. However, don't go too far and starve yourself. If you don't want to start your morning bike on an empty stomach, eat an hour or so before you ride.

SWIMMING

Swimming may not be your first thinking when it comes to losing weight. Are you curious about the potential benefits of swimming for weight loss? Does it really work?

Yes, it is a resounding yes. Swimming provides a total-body workout.

If you enjoy swimming or have tried other forms of exercise with little success, we're about to dive (pun intended) into everything you need to know about swimming for weight loss, including how many calories you can burn and the best swimming routines to help you achieve a healthy weight.

Is swimming useful for losing weight?
Swimming is sometimes misunderstood as ineffective for weight loss. There are individuals who claim that strolling around a pool is more advantageous than actually swimming in it.

However, research suggests otherwise. Swimming and walking were both practiced at the same intensity and frequency (3 times per week) in one study to examine their impact on weight loss. When compared to the walking group, the swimming group shed 2 pounds and 0.7 inches from their waistline.

Swimming may be worth exploring if you're trying to lose weight and haven't found joy in running, strength training, or going to the gym. Swimming, like any other workout, burns calories because the water offers resistance.

Swimming also trains every part of your body at the same time, from your upper body to your lower body and core.

According to a 2015 study, women who swam for an hour three times a week reported significant reductions in belly fat, improvements in flexibility and strength, and even a fall in cholesterol levels.

How does swimming aid with weight loss?

Swimming is a full-body workout that engages many muscles in your body. Specific body areas are targeted by various strokes such as the butterfly, breaststroke, and backstroke. The butterfly and breaststroke work the chest, arms, and shoulders, whereas the backstroke works the abs, back, and quadriceps.

Furthermore, because swimming is a water-based exercise, the water generates resistance, which your body's strength is needed to overcome.

Swimming is also far better for your joints than running or walking, lowering your risk of injury and boosting your chances of regular activity, which benefits in weight reduction.

How far do you have to swim in order to lose weight?
Consistency and maintaining a calorie deficit are the keys to losing weight regardless of exercise.

When it comes to losing weight, some people argue that what you eat is actually more crucial than the amount of physical activity you engage in. So, if you're eating poorly and swimming to lose weight, it won't make much of a difference.

To burn calories when swimming, both the duration and intensity of your swim exercise are important. Swimming at a moderate intensity for an hour can burn up to 500 calories.
Changing your swimming strokes can also help you burn more calories.

Another way to burn more calories when swimming is to shorten your rest times. Swimming for longer periods of time and resting less frequently keeps your heart rate up and helps you burn more calories.

How many calories do you burn while you swim?
The number of calories expended during a swimming session is determined by the intensity of your workout. Swimming activities can burn up to 800 calories per hour. If you swim four times per week, you should expect to lose 2-4 pounds per month.

A half-hour moderate-intensity workout burns roughly 250 calories if you're just starting out with swimming and gradually rising from low to high intensity. If you do this four times each week, you should expect to lose one pound per month.

It's also worth noting that calorie burn differs from individual to person. The calories burned are impacted by your present weight and the intensity with which you swim, according to Harvard Health.

Individuals weighing 125 pounds can burn 180 calories in a 30-minute swimming exercise at a moderate speed, whereas those weighing 154 pounds can burn 216 calories and those weighing 182 pounds can burn 252 calories.

Those weighing 125 pounds may burn 300 calories in a strenuous 30-minute swimming session, those weighing 154 pounds can burn 360 calories, and those weighing 182 pounds can burn 420 calories.

What is the best weight-loss swimming routine?

If you've never tried swimming for weight reduction before, it may be good to begin with a mild effort and progressively raise your intensity.

## REAPING REWARDS AND CELEBRATING SUCCESS

There are numerous advantages to losing weight. You can enhance your physical health, lower your risk of chronic diseases, and boost your energy levels by losing excess weight. Improvements in your mental health, such as enhanced self-confidence and a more optimistic view on life, may also be noticed.

Additionally, losing weight can contribute to better sleep, digestion, and a stronger immune system. Not to mention the thrill of once again fitting into your favorite outfits! So, by committing to a healthy lifestyle and meeting your weight loss objectives, you may reap all of these wonderful benefits and live a happier, healthier life.

Sometimes real rewards are required along the way to keep you motivated and to celebrate big milestones. It's like a carrot dangling in front of you. (In fact, toss out the whole idea of food as a reward!)

According to Abby Langer, an expert in food and nutrition from Canada, incorporating non-food incentives or rewards can be an enjoyable method to maintain people's motivation towards achieving their weight loss objectives. "However, I noted the emphasis on 'non-food.' In general, it's not a good idea to use food as a reward or punishment."

The battle is great when it comes to clothing yourself while reducing weight. Buying a new pair of designer jeans every time you go down a size may not be feasible.

However, gym clothes that don't have to be form-fitting and high-quality yoga pants are a smart investment while you're losing weight. Furthermore, being comfortable and looking nice are too strong temptations to continue.

Getting a Massage:

Give your body a pleasant massage. Massage therapy not only feels nice, but it can also enhance blood flow and heal tight muscles, according to a study published in the Archives of Physical Medicine and Rehabilitation by the University of Illinois at Chicago.

Another study conducted by the University of Alabama at Birmingham discovered that massage therapy can help lower blood pressure, prevent colds, and even improve skin tone. So schedule your massage right away!

Getting a Pedicure:

And these piglets went to the salon! This is an especially good idea for anyone whose feet have been working hard to help them reduce weight. (Looking at you, joggers and walkers!) Aside from the esthetic benefits of having well-kept toes, a pedicure can provide moisture to your feet, preventing them from breaking. Brissette suggests turning it into a spa day with a massage or manicure if you can afford it. With enthusiasm, she exclaims, "You've earned it for all your diligent efforts!"

Flowers:

Although you certainly didn't need a study to tell you that flowers can help individuals feel happier and more energetic, Harvard researchers discovered. However, to master this happiness hack, place the flowers on your nightstand.

The Harvard researchers, who worked in collaboration with Massachusetts General Hospital, were able to confirm that those who did not consider themselves "morning people" experienced a happiness boost gazing at the blossoms right at sunrise, observing them as the day began.

A Lunch Container:

According to a 2013 study published in BMJ, the average adult takeout meal has 836 calories. Yowza! If you packed your own 500-calorie lunch, you'd save 1,680 calories during the work week. But, let's face it: your brown paper lunch bag is a little depressing. It could also be holding you back. Upgrade to a lunch pack with insulated cooler bags and better storage for your Tupperware and cutlery.

Elegant Water Bottle:

Having your own specific water container, whether it's a Swell bottle or a Camelbak, makes sipping water throughout the day that much easier.

A study published in The Journal of Clinical Endocrinology and Metabolism indicated that drinking water can be beneficial to your metabolism. Drinking 17 ounces of water resulted in a 30% rise in metabolic rate across participants!

Subscription to a Fitness or Healthy Eating Magazine:

Your inbox has been consuming a lot of garbage (mail). Complement its diet by subscribing to a fitness magazine or any other publication focusing on good life.

Flipping through a glossy magazine is entertaining!

Furthermore, it could be the motivation you need to attempt a new meal, yoga posture, or activity. Magazines.com has a ton of excellent prices on great titles.

# CONCLUSION

"Congratulations on taking the first step toward a healthier and happier you!" This book has given you all of the tools and knowledge you need to reach your weight loss objectives. So, start adopting these suggestions and watch your body and mind transform.

You deserve to feel fantastic, and this book will assist you in getting there!

Exploring "Slim Down Revolution" allows us to regain control of our eating patterns and make informed decisions for ourselves.

We may improve our relationship with food and uncover the best version of ourselves by following the concepts taught in this book.

It's a call to prioritize our well-being, adopt a healthy lifestyle, and realize our full potential.

In summary, "Slim Down Revolution" is an invaluable resource that simplifies weight loss, allows us to unlock our inner health, and guides us to becoming the best version of ourselves.
Let us go on this enlightening adventure together in order to create a better, happier future.

## FINAL THOUGHTS AND ENCOURAGEMENT

The book "Slim Down Revolution" is a powerful resource that aims to guide individuals on their journey towards achieving a healthier and more balanced lifestyle. As we reach the end of this transformative book, it is important to reflect on the key takeaways and offer some final thoughts and encouragement.

First and foremost, congratulations on taking the initiative to embark on this revolution towards a slimmer and healthier you. Recognizing the need for change and taking action is a significant step in itself. Throughout the book, you have gained valuable insights into nutrition, exercise, mindset, and other essential aspects of weight loss and overall well-being.

Remember that the journey towards a healthier lifestyle is not a quick fix or a temporary solution. It is a lifelong commitment to making sustainable changes that will benefit your physical and mental health in the long run. Embrace the principles and strategies outlined in "Slim Down Revolution" as a foundation for your ongoing journey.

It is important to approach your goals with patience and kindness towards yourself. Weight loss and lifestyle changes can be challenging, and setbacks are a natural part of the process. Don't be discouraged by temporary obstacles or plateaus. Instead, view them as opportunities for growth and learning. Stay focused on your long-term vision and celebrate every small victory along the way.

Surround yourself with a supportive network of friends, family, or even online communities who share similar goals. Having a support system can provide encouragement, accountability, and motivation during times when you may feel discouraged or tempted to revert to old habits. Share your progress, seek advice, and offer support to others on their own journeys.

Lastly, remember that self-care goes beyond just physical health. Take time to nurture your mental and emotional well-being. Practice self-compassion, engage in activities that bring you joy, and prioritize rest and relaxation. Remember that a healthy lifestyle is not just about the number on the scale but also about feeling energized, confident, and fulfilled.

As you conclude your reading of "Slim Down Revolution," carry the knowledge and inspiration gained from this book into your daily life. Embrace the power of small, consistent steps towards your goals, and believe in your ability to create lasting change. You have the tools and the determination to make a positive impact on your health and well-being. Best of luck on your continued journey towards a healthier, happier you!

www.ingramcontent.com/pod-product-compliance
Lightning Source LLC
Chambersburg PA
CBHW060945260726
48661CB00005B/1770